KETO PIZZA

Discover 30 Easy to Follow Ketogenic Cookbook Pizza recipes for Your Low-Carb Diet with Gluten-Free and wheat to Maximize your weight loss

STEPHANIE BAKER

Copyright © Stephanie Baker

All rights reserved. No part of this book may be reproduced, scanned or distributed in any printed or electronic form without permission. Please do not participate in or encourage piracy of copyrighted materials in violation of the author's rights. Purchase only authorized editions.

1
LOW CARB PIZZA

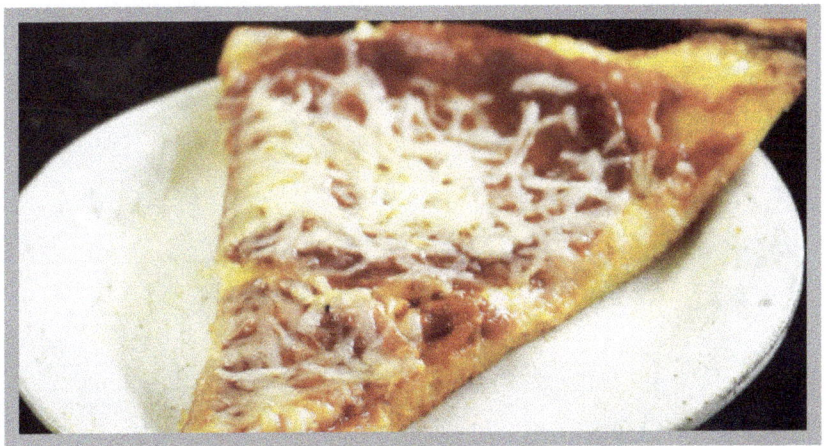

20 MINUTES.
  Easy
  893 kcal

INGREDIENTS

1 servings

- 1 half can of tuna in its own juice
- 3 eggs)
- 2 slices of cooked ham
- 1 ½ teaspoon of heaped tomato paste
- N.b. Salt and pepper
- N. B. Topping for oregano or pizza
- 80 g of grated cheese

NUTRITIONAL VALUES per serving

Kcal

893

Protein

113.41 g

Fat

45.52 g

Carbohydrate

6.38 g

PREPARATION

1. Processing time about 20 minutes
2. Cooking / cooking time approx. 30 minutes.
3. Total time about 50 minutes
4. First put the tuna in a colander over a bowl, tear it and drain it. Mix two eggs in a bowl, add the drained

tuna, mix everything with a fork, then knead with your hands.

1. Lightly grease a pizza pan and line the bottom with parchment paper. Alternatively, you can use a normal oven tray.

1. Now spread the egg and tuna mixture evenly on top and press it with a spoon until it forms a pizza base about 1/2 centimeter high. Now bake the base for 10-15 minutes at 180 °c and a convection of 160 °c.

1. Meanwhile, cut the ham into small pieces. Place 1.5 teaspoons of tomato paste on the cooked base and distribute evenly. Spread over the cooked ham.
2. Sprinkle everything with pepper, salt and lots of seasoning for the pizza, alternatively oregano, and spread the grated cheese on top. Put the egg in the center.

1. Bake pizza at the same temperature for another 15-20 minutes.

2

THE BEST AND SIMPLEST LOW CARB PIZZA WITH CREAM CHEESE, CHEESE AND EGG BASE

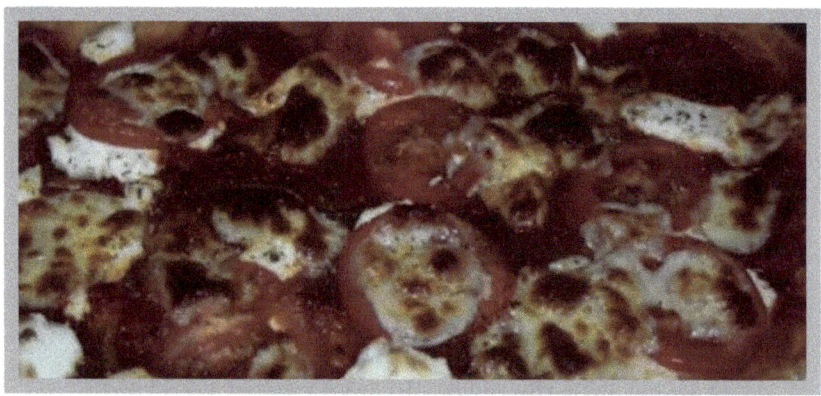

10 MINUTES.
   Normal

INGREDIENTS
   2 servings
   For the floor:

- 4 eggs)
- 200 g of grated cheese
- 150 g of cream cheese

Cover:

- 100 g of seasoned tomato sauce
- 100 g of grated mozzarella
- N.b. Vegetables and / or mushrooms
- N.b. Salami or ham or other condiments

PREPARATION

1. Processing time about 10 minutes.
2. Cooking / cooking time about 40 minutes
3. Total time about 50 minutes
4. Preheat the oven to 180 ° c.

1. Mix the cream cheese and eggs in a bowl with a whisk. Then add the grated cheese and mix well. Distribute the mixture evenly on the pan; parchment paper is recommended. Beware, the dough is still relatively liquid but will become firmer after cooking.

1. Bake in the oven for about 30 minutes until golden

brown. Then garnish the base with the tomato sauce, desired toppings and mozzarella. Put it in the oven for another 10 minutes.

1. Low carb pizza is very similar to real pizza and contains only 9g of carbs.

3
LOW CARB PIZZA PRAWN

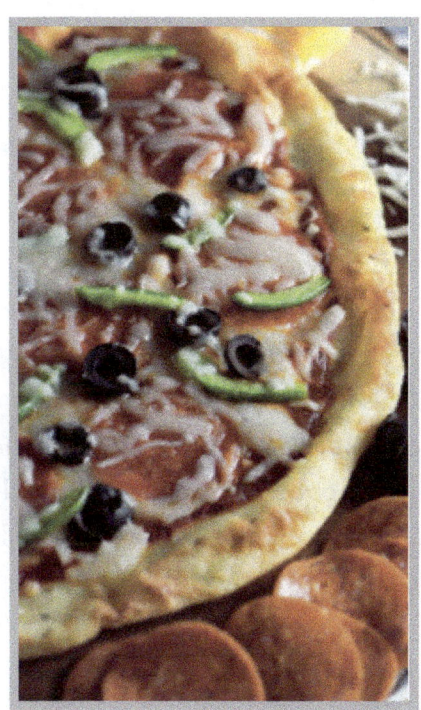

15 MINUTES.

Normal

INGREDIENTS

2 servings

- 1 ½ can of tuna in its own juice
- 3 eggs)
- 2 slices of cooked ham
- 80 g of grated cheese of your choice
- Salt and pepper
- Origan
- Ketchup

PREPARATION

1. Processing time about 15 minutes
2. Cooking time / cooking approx. 35 minutes.
3. Total time about 50 minutes
4. Mix two eggs well in a bowl. Drain the tuna, add it to the eggs and mix everything well. Place the mixture on a baking sheet of parchment paper and shape it into a round shape. The background should be approximately 0.4-0.6cm thick. Cook the bottom of the tuna for 10-15 minutes at 180 ° c high / low in a preheated oven.

1. Then take out of the oven, spread with tomato sauce and season with salt, pepper and oregano. Break the slices of ham and cover them with the pizza. Sprinkle with cheese, break the third egg and place it on the pizza.

1. Then put the pizza back in the oven and cook for about 20 minutes, until the egg has solidified and the cheese has a nice golden color.

1. Obviously, the pizza can also be coated differently as desired.

4
LOW CARB CAULIFLOWER PIZZA BASE

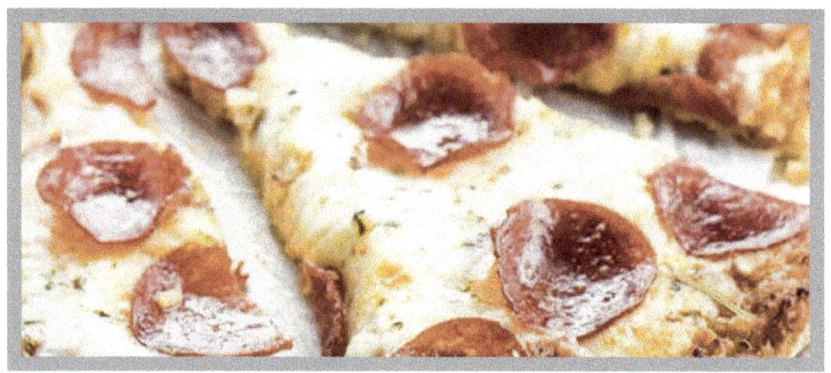

30 minutes.

Easy

INGREDIENTS
2 servings

- Approx. 250 g cauliflower, cooked and chopped
- 200 g grated cheese, preferably light
- 1 egg (s)
- 1 teaspoon of freshly chopped garlic
- ½ teaspoon of garlic salt
- 1 teaspoon of aromatic herbs, italian of your choice
- A little olive oil if possible
- North. B. Pizza sauce

PREPARATION

1. Working time approx. 30 minutes
2. Cooking time / cooking time approx. 30 minutes
3. Total time approx. 1 hour
4. Remove all the stems and leaves from the cauliflower and cut the cabbage into small pieces. Chop in the food processor until it looks like parmesan. If you don't have a food processor, you can also try it with a grater, a sharp knife (shave the whole head) or a magic wand (but not too thick, it shouldn't be puree).

1. Place the chopped cauliflower in a microwave-safe bowl and cook for about 8 minutes. No need to addin water as the natural moisture is sufficient. How to do it when you don't have a microwave i don't know. I suspect it can work with thawed frozen cabbage or

pre-cooked cabbage as well. So i didn't have enough testing options.

1. A large cauliflower makes 3 to 4 "cups" (about 250 ml per cup). A pizza cup is required for 2-3 people. The remaining dough from the cabbage crumb can be stored in the refrigerator for up to 1 week.

1. Set the oven to approx. 230 ° c. Line a tray with parchment paper or parchment paper. In a bowl, 1 cup (approx. 200 g) cauliflower, an egg and approx. 200 g of grated cheese. Then there are the herbs, garlic, and salt.

1. Mix everything vigorously. This should simply be a pulp. At first i thought it might never work ... After all, it's a completely different consistency from sourdough, but because of these doubts we just have to move on.

1. Roll out the dough on the pan and roll it out with your hands in the shape and thickness you want. If you really want, you can brush the surface with olive

oil to promote browning. Bake at 230 °c for about 15 minutes (until it's deliciously golden).

1. Take out of the oven and spread with pizza sauce. Then cover as desired (but do not use raw ground beef, as the pizza is now only cooked). Put everything back in the oven for about 10 minutes, until the cheese is melted or golden yellow.

5
LOW CARB PIZZA TRIANGLE

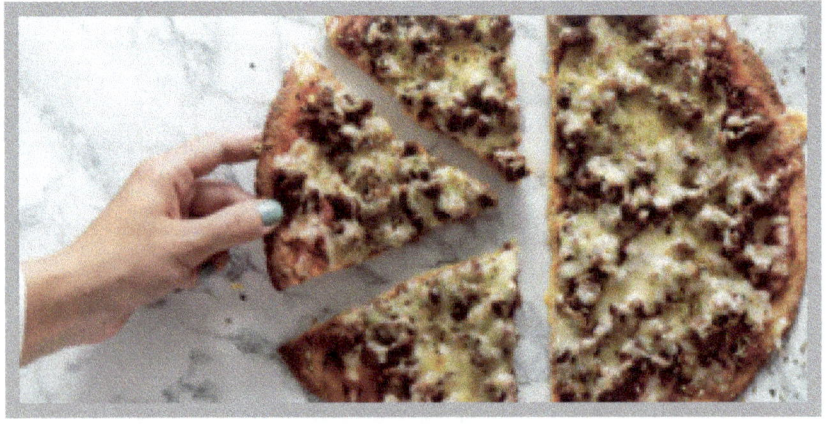

15 MINUTES.
   Easy
   1102 kcal

INGREDIENTS

KETO PIZZA

1 servings

- 1 can of tuna in its own juice
- 200 g of cottage cheese
- 2 eggs)
- 1 tablespoon cheese (hard cheese), grated
- 3 tablespoons of wheat bran

Nutritional values per serving
Kcal
1102
Protein
80.22 g
Fat
84.13 g
Carbohydrate
6.78 g

PREPARATION

1. Working time approx. 15 minutes
2. Cooking time / cooking time approx. 35 minutes
3. Total time approx. 50 minutes
4. Preheat the oven to 180 degrees of air circulation.

1. Drain the tuna well and place in a bowl with all the

other ingredients. Beat everything as gently as possible with a fork. Then use a fork to press the dough onto a parchment-lined baking sheet for a pizza crust.

1. Then place the bottom in the oven on a top rack for 30-35 minutes and cook.

1. Then you can cover the dough with the pizza sauce and, if you like, sprinkle basil, chorizo or vegetables with mozzarella or parmesan and put back in the oven to cook until the cheese turns color and melts.

6
LOW CARB PIZZA YVES

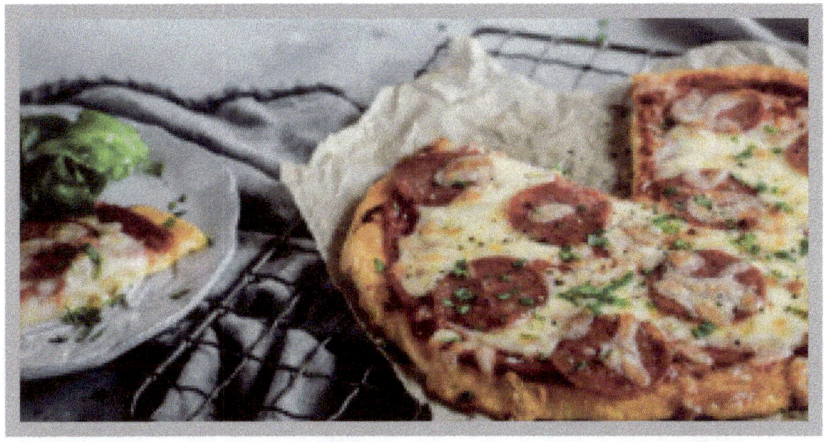

45 MIN.
 Normal

728 kcal

. . .

INGREDIENTS

4 servings

- 200 g quark
- 3 eggs)
- 180 g cheese (gouda or mozzarella)
- 1 cup of fresh cream cheese
- 200 g mixed cheese for gratinating
- ½ chives)
- 250 g mushrooms, brown
- 3 peppers, red, yellow, green
- 250 g ham
- Salt and pepper
- Origan

Nutritional values per serving
Kcal
728
Protein
52.18 g
Fat
52.68 g
Carbohydrate
11.11 g

PREPARATION

1. Working time approx. 45 minutes

2. Cooking time / cooking time approx. 30 minutes
3. Total time approx. 1 hour and 15 minutes
4. All ingredients are intended for a baking sheet.

1. Preheat the oven to 180 degrees.

1. Cut the vegetables and ham into thin strips.

1. For the batter, mix the cottage cheese, eggs, and spices into a smooth mixture, then add the grated cheese. Place the parchment paper on a baking sheet and roll out the dough on it. Approx. 15 minutes, middle track (upper / lower heat).

1. Take the pre-cooked dough out of the oven and let it cool slightly. Then spread the fresh cream on the dough and garnish with chives, ham, mushrooms and paprika. Then sprinkle the rest of the cheese on top and cook for another 15 minutes.

7
LOW CARB PIZZA WITH SAUCE

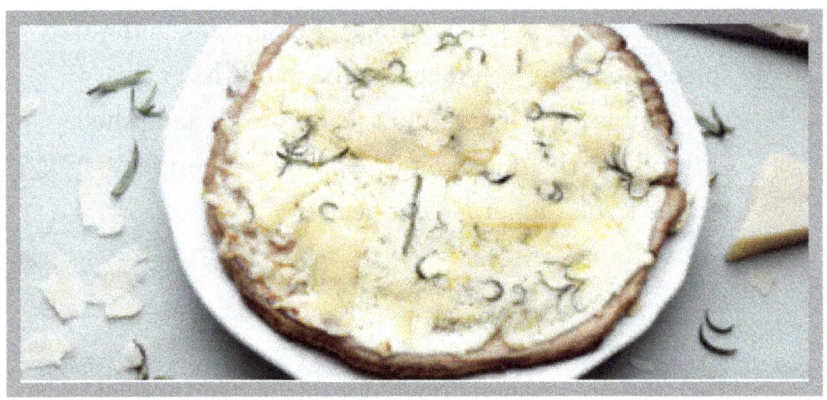

30 MINUTES.
   Normal

INGREDIENTS
   Two portions
   For pasta:

- 2 cans / n of tuna in its own juice
- 2 tablespoons full ricotta or granulated cream cheese
- 2 eggs)
- For the sauce:
- 200 ml of tomatoes passed
- Salt-
- Pepper
- Origan
- For the filling: for example
- 1 bell pepper
- 1 zucchini
- 3 slices of cooked ham
- Some corn
- Similarity:

SOME GRATED CHEESE

PREPARATION

1. Processing time of about 30 minutes.
2. Rest time of about 5 minutes.
3. Cooking / cooking time approx. 35 minutes
4. Total time about 1 hour and 10 minutes.
5. For the batter, first drain the tuna well and put it in a bowl, then add the ricotta and the 2 eggs and mix everything well. The best way to do this is with a fork.

1. If the tuna batter is well mixed and doughy, you've done everything right and can now spread it evenly over the pan. Preferably with a fork so you can flatten it evenly. Don't be too skinny though, otherwise everything will fall apart later!

1. Now the dough is put in a preheated oven at 180 ° c for 10-15 minutes.

1. Meanwhile, you can prepare the sauce and other ingredients with which you want to decorate your pizza.

1. For the sauce, i put the tomatoes in a small bowl, seasoned them, and mixed them with salt, pepper, and oregano.

1. Then cut the other ingredients into small pieces or strips for the garnish. I slicedthe zucchini and pan-fried them before covering.

1. When the dough is ready you can take it out of the oven, let it rest for 5 minutes and then spread the tomato sauce finely.

1. Next, put some grated cheese on top of the tomato sauce so the topping doesn't fall off and the base connects to the pizza topping.

1. Now you can decorate your pizza to your liking. For me it was cooked ham, peppers, zucchini, and corn.

1. In the last step, sprinkle the pizza with cheese and then bake it for 15-20 minutes at 180 ° c.

8
LOW CARB EGGPLANT PIZZA

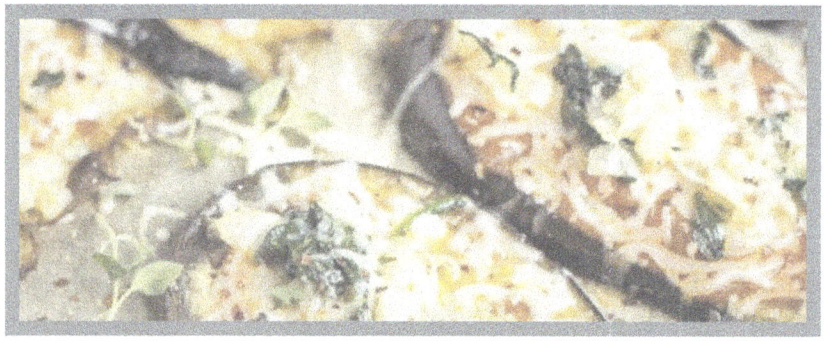

50 MIN.
Normal
508 kcal

INGREDIENTS
4 portions

- 40g butter
- 250 ml of tomatoes passed
- 100 g of cooked ham
- 100g paprika sausage (pepper salami), spicy
- 250 g middle-aged gouda cheese
- 100 g of mushrooms
- Topping for pizza or oregano
- Salt and pepper
- Paprika powder
- Eggplants, about 250 g each

Nutritional values per serving
Kcal
508
Protein
30.94 g
Fat
37.37 g
Carbohydrate
12.02 g

PREPARATION

1. Processing time of about 50 minutes.
2. Rest time about 1 hour.
3. Cooking / cooking time approx. 25 minutes
4. Total time about 2 hours and 15 minutes.
5. Wash and pat the aubergines and remove the stem.

Cut each eggplant into 5 slices, preferably with an electric slicer. Set the 3 middle slices aside and use elsewhere. Sprinkle the two slightly bulbous outer slices over the cut surface with salt and leave covered for at least 1 hour.

1. Do not dry the wet aubergines and place them on a baking sheet cut surface down. Pour 100 ml of water and cook in a hot oven at 200 ° c for about 20 minutes. When the water has evaporated after 10 minutes, add again 100ml of water if necessary. Take off the aubergines from the oven and allow to cool slightly.

1. Now line the pan with parchment paper and place the eggplants with the covered skin next to each other in the pan.

1. Melt the butter and put it in a large bowl. Mix with the tomatoes. Cut the ham, the paprika salami and the mushrooms into cubes and add them. Finely grate the cheese and about 200 g. Season the mixture with pizza toppings or other toppings as needed. If the pizza mix istoo runny, add a little more shredded cheese.

1. Put about 50g of pizza mix on each of the aubergines and bake at 180-200 °c for about 25 minutes.

1. The pizza mix, of course, can also be made with other toppings like tuna, onions, olives, whatever you want on the pizza. The amount of cheese is necessary for the joint, otherwise the dough will flow too much during cooking.

1. The center aubergine slices left here can also be salted, dried, brushed with herb oil and fried until golden brown or placed on the grill. I have not tested if the middle slices can also be used as a pizza eggplant. I thought the side discs with the casing were better because they are stronger and will not flake.

9
LOW CARB CHEESE PIZZA

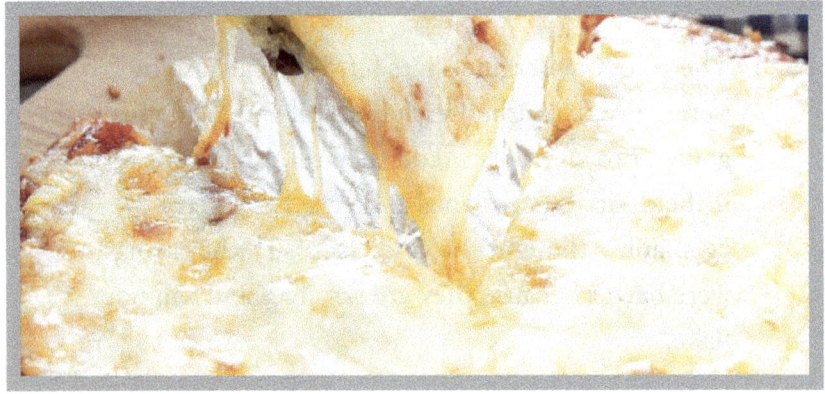

20 MINUTES.
Easy
525 kcal

INGREDIENTS
4 servings

- 200 g cream cheese plus granules
- 4th egg / 1.
- 50 g of chopped almonds
- 1 pepper, red or yellow
- 200 g cooked ham
- 200 g of grated cheese
- 1 small red onion
- 150 g turkey breast in pieces or strips
- 50 g diced ham
- Salt and pepper
- Origan

Nutritional values per serving

Kcal

525

Protein

50.92 g

Fat

33.12 g

Carbohydrate

5.68 g

PREPARATION

1. Working time approx. 20 minutes
2. Cooking time / cooking time approx. 20 minutes
3. Total time approx. 40 minutes
4. Cut the onion, bell pepper, ham and turkey breast to

the required size.

1. Inside a bowl with a whisk, mix the wholemeal cream cheese with the chopped eggs and almonds. Only then add paprika, ham and spices and mix everything well. Finally add the grated cheese.

1. Now distribute the whole mixture on a baking sheet. It is better to put a sheet of parchment paper under it, sticking out a little on all sides. This way you can easily take the pizza out of the pan later.

1. Now spread the onions, diced ham and strips of turkey breast on the pizza base and bake the pizza at 200 degrees for about 20-25 minutes. The edge can get very dark.

LOW CARB, HIGH PROTEIN PIZZA

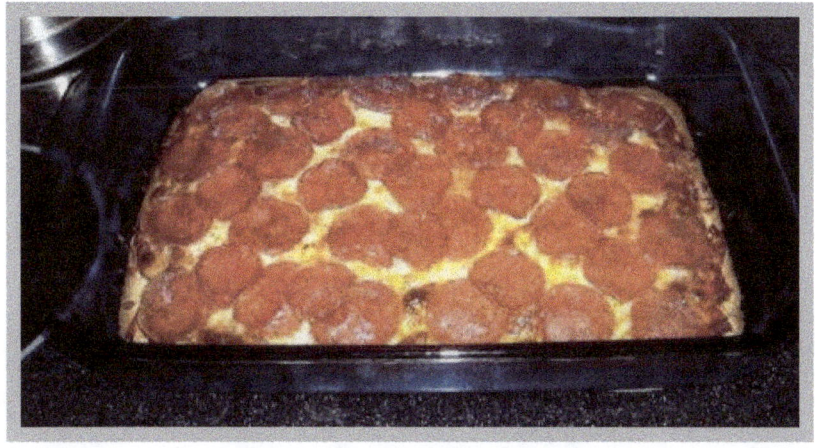

10 MINS.
   Easy
   520 kcal

INGREDIENTS

1 servings

- 1 large egg
- 1 can of tuna
- 2 slices of chicken breast fillets
- 5 small slice (noun) salami (chicken salami)
- 1 m. Of large tomatoes)
- 20 g jalapeños
- 40 g lightly baked cheese
- 20 g tomato paste
- Herbs
- Salt and pepper

PREPARATION

1. Working time approx. 10 minutes
2. Cooking time / cooking time approx. 30 minutes
3. Total time approx. 40 minutes
4. First mix the egg with the can of tuna and mix with a little salt and pepper. Spread evenly on a baking sheet lined with parchment paper and bake at approx. 200 ° c. 10-15 minutes.

1. Then mix the tomato paste with a dash of water, salt, pepper and some aromatic herbs of your choice and spread them over the base of the finished pizza.

1. Fill it to taste (in my example with salami, chicken, tomato, jalapeños and cheese) and then put it back in the oven for about 15 minutes at 200 ° c.

1. In my example, the whole pizza is only 520 kcal.

1. Low carb pancakes, crepes, wrap, pizza, pancake batter

FIVE MINUTES PIZZA

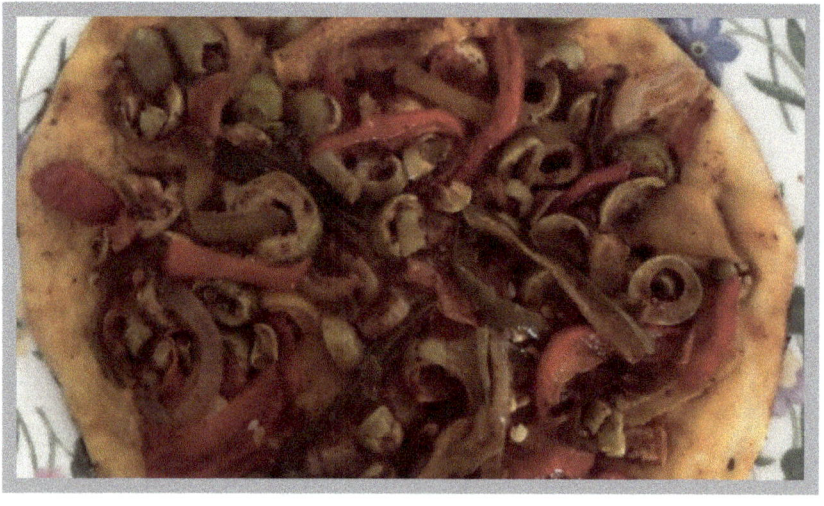

Normal
207 kcal

INGREDIENTS

2 servings
Fourth protein

- 500 ml buttermilk
- 30 g psyllium husks, ground
- 45 g coconut flour
- 1 teaspoon of baking powder
- 1 pinch of salt

NUTRITIONAL VALUES per serving
Kcal
207
Protein
21.40 g
Fat
4.03 g
Carbohydrate
14.06 g

PREPARATION

1. Working time approx. Five minutes
2. Rest time approx. 10 minutes
3. Cooking time / cooking time approx. 30 minutes
4. Total time approx. 45 minutes
5. This universal low-carbohydrate dough can be used for almost anything. It is also ideal for further processing when it is unseasoned and tasteless.

1. Mix all the ingredients until you get a homogeneous mixture. At first it is still a little runny, but as soon as the psyllium husks have swollen a little, they can be processed.

1. Let the dough soak for about 10 minutes.

1. Depending on the consistency of the coconut flour, it can be too fine or too thick. So add a little more or less coconut flour or buttermilk. However, you should try a few times and give only a little after the swelling. However, it was perfect for me with coconut fiber flour and the stated amounts.

1. After the puffing phase, roll out the relatively thin dough on a baking sheet lined with parchment paper and place it with a fan in the oven preheated to 180 ° c for about 30 minutes. Cooking times can change due to oven to oven and the dough should be light. The dough inflates like a balloon, but as soon as the oven door opens or cools, it slowly collapses again. Therefore no drilling is required.

1. After cooling, the dough is very pliable and flexible and can be put back in the oven with a pizza topping, rolled up like a foil or filled like a sweet or savory pancake.

1. I like the sweet version best with a little vanilla in the batter and a quark spread with fresh fruit or fruit, but also the savory version as a wrap with garlic and oregano in the batter, filled with cherry tomatoes, rocket, delicious mozzarella, chicken and pesto.

1. The whole dough has about 340 kcal and is thick enough for 2 strong guests. So you have around 170 kcal per person without coverage.

12

LOW CARB PIZZA MADE FROM CREAM CHEESE DOUGH

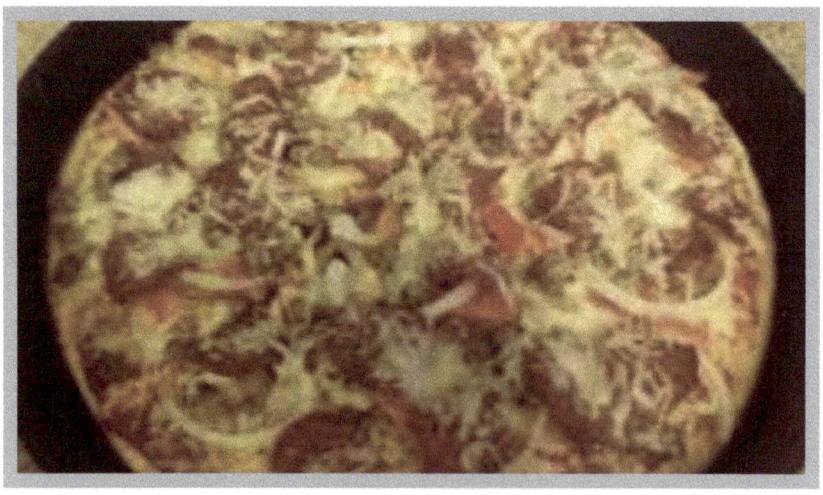

10 MINS.

Easy

. . .

KETO PIZZA

INGREDIENTS

2 servings

- 3 eggs)
- 100 g cream cheese
- 2 tablespoons of almond flour
- 1 pinch of baking powder
- 1 heaped teaspoon of salt
- 1 teaspoon of oregano

PREPARATION

1. Processing time approx. 10 minutes
2. Cooking time / cooking time approx. 45 minutes
3. Total time approx. 55 minutes
4. Mix the ingredients, season well and arrange on a baking sheet (the dough is almost runny). Now bake at 180 ° c for about 30 minutes.

1. When the time is up, turn the base over, puncture the batter, garnish with tomato sauce and ingredients of your choice, and put it back in the oven until it suits you.

1. The dough will be compact, you can cut it right into the corners. However, it won't get as crispy as you know it from the normal crust.

1. I think it's a great alternative to real dough. I don't miss the old pizza.

13
FAST LOW CARB PIZZA

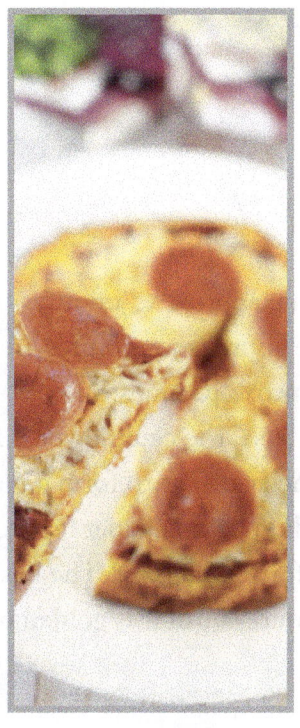

10 MINS.

Normal

INGREDIENTS

1 servings

- 2 eggs)
- 200 g cauliflower
- Possibly. Ham
- Possibly. Mozzarella cheese
- 2 tablespoons of tomato paste
- 50 g tomato (s), chopped from the can
- 1 teaspoon of oregano
- ½ clove of garlic)

PREPARATION

1. Processing time approx. 10 minutes
2. Cooking time approx. 30 minutes
3. Total time approx. 40 minutes
4. For the pizza base, the cauliflower is finely grated and mixed with the two eggs to form a mass.
5. This is spread on baking paper (approx. 0.5 cm - 1 cm thick) in the form of a pizza. The base is baked at 220 ° for 15-20 minutes until it is golden on the surface.

1. For the pizza sauce, mix the tomato paste, half a clove of garlic, oregano and chopped tomatoes well and place on the golden brown pizza crust.
2. If you want, you can now add mozzarella, ham, or similar ingredients to the pizza.
3. Put in the oven for another 10 minutes.

1. Tip: the pizza is likely to be stuck on parchment paper. To loosen it is turned over with parchment paper and the parchment paper can be easily peeled off.

14
LOW CARB ZUCCHINI PIZZA

KETO PIZZA

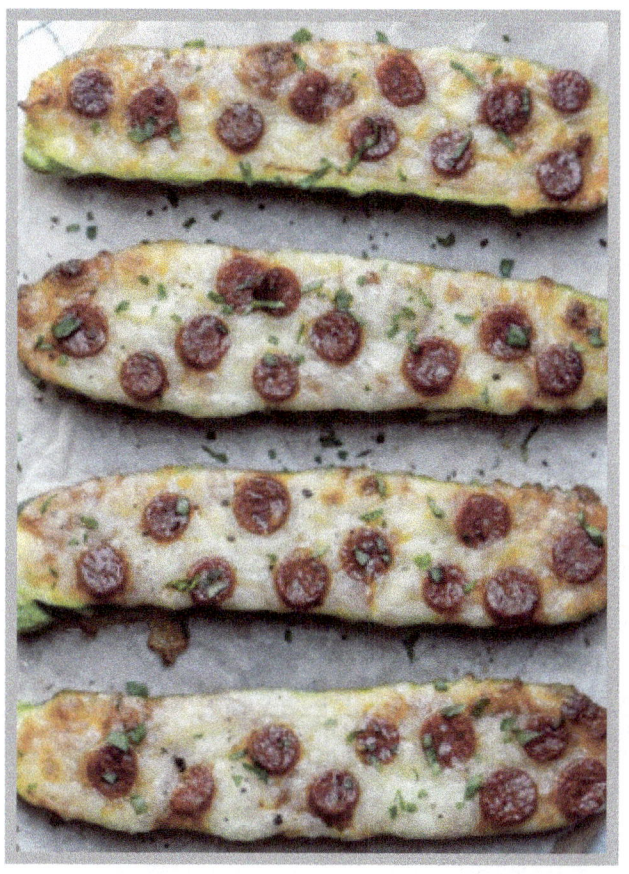

20 MINUTES.

Normal

INGREDIENTS

1 servings

- 2 m zucchini
- 100 g grated mozzarella
- 2 eggs)

- Cocktail tomatoes
- 1 tablespoon of mozzarella, sliced
- 2 tablespoons of tomato sauce
- 1 teaspoon of oregano
- 1 teaspoon of salt
- 1 teaspoon of pepper
- Fresh basil

PREPARATION

1. Processing time approx. 20 minutes
2. Cooking time approx. 30 minutes
3. Total time approx. 50 minutes
4. Wash the zucchini, rub them, put them in a cloth, wrap them well and squeeze them so that they squeeze out as much water as possible.

1. Put the drained rasps in a bowl, add the eggs, grated cheese, salt and pepper and mix well. Line a baking sheet with parchment paper. Spread the zucchini mixture over it and use the spoon to form a round pizza base. The bottom should not be thicker than 1/2 cm. Bake in the oven at 220 °c for about 20 minutes.

1. Take out the bottom and z. Cover with mozzarella, tomatoes and basil, for example. Scatter oregano on top. Set the oven on the highest temperature for 5 - 10 minutes and make sure nothing burns.

1. Cut and serve.

15
LOW-CARB CESROLE

KETO PIZZA

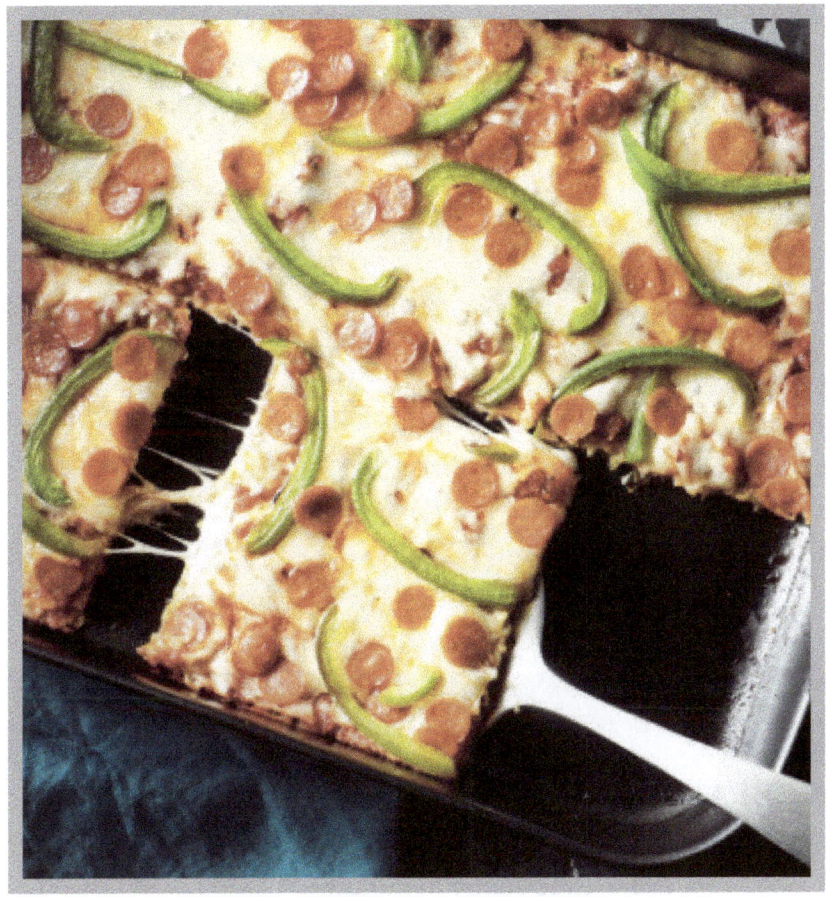

10 MIN.

Normal

2433 kcal

INGREDIENTS

1 portions

- 600 g of head
- 5 egg (s), measure. M.

- 500 g of grated cheese
- 2 tablespoons of chia seeds nb
- A little bit of salt

Nutritional values per serving

Kcal

2433

Protein

160.95 g

Fat

191.25 g

Carbohydrate

14.09 g

PREPARATION

1. Processing time about 10 minutes
2. Rest time about 10 minutes
3. Cooking time / cooking approx. 25 minutes
4. Total time about 45 minutes
5. Preheat the oven to 160 ° c.

1. Wash the cauliflower florets (like a large cauliflower) and drain very well. You shouldn't be wet anymore. Then rub to form the grain size of the rice grains. Now all the ingredients (chia seeds remove some

moisture from the dough) are mixed with a wooden spoon and spread on a baking sheet lined with parchment paper. When the chia seeds have been processed, let the mixture rest for 10 minutes before spreading it on the parchment paper.

1. Then bake the dough for about 25-30 minutes.

1. If desired, further process the base, i.e. For example as a topping for pizza or as a flambé cake. Then bake for another 10-15 minutes.

16
LOW CARB PIZZA BOAT

KETO PIZZA

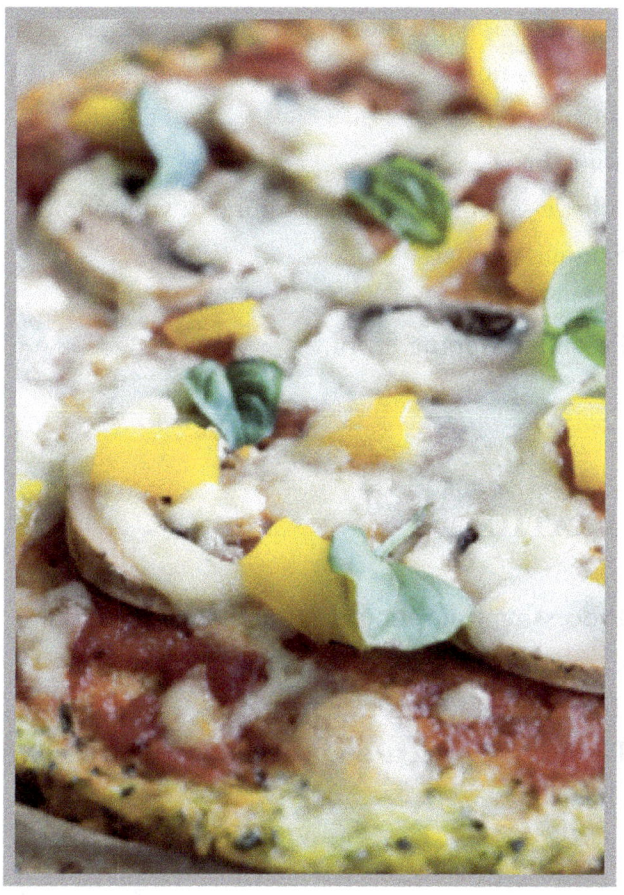

5 MINUTES.
   Easy

INGREDIENTS
   4 servings

- 300 g of cottage cheese
- 120 g of grated cheese
- 3 eggs)

- 25 g of chopped almonds
- A little onion
- A little pepper
- Some ham
- A little salami or other seasoning of your choice
- Salt and pepper
- Possibly. Basil
- Possibly. Topping for pizza

PREPARATION

1. Processing time about 5 minutes
2. Cooking / cooking time approx. 30 minutes
3. Total time about 35 minutes
4. Preheat the oven to 200 ° c pre-air. Prepare a baking sheet.

1. Combine the ricotta, grated cheese, eggs and chopped almonds in a bowl. Spread on the pan and season.

1. Top with the dressing if desired and bake in the oven for about 20-30 minutes.

17

LOW-CARB MINCED PIZZA

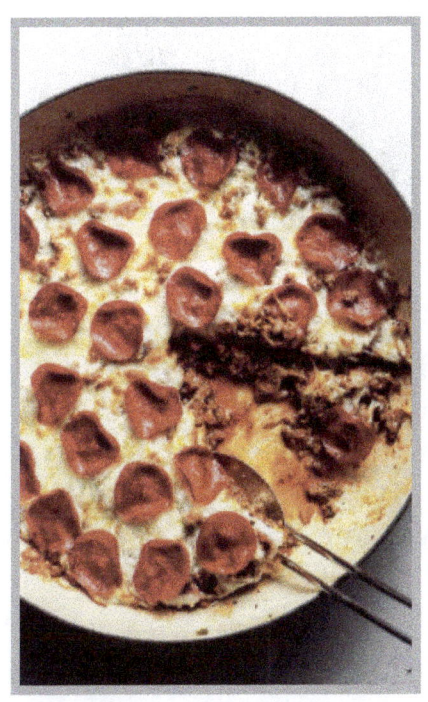

30 MINUTES.

Normal
693 kcal

INGREDIENTS
8 servings

- 1 ½ kg of minced meat, mixed
- 375 g of tomato (s) have passed
- 200 g of grated mozzarella
- 75 g of sour cream
- 50 ml of water
- 3 onion (noun)
- 3 cloves of garlic)
- 3 peppers
- 1 bunch of chives (m)
- 2 eggs)
- 1 tablespoon of tomato paste
- 2 tablespoons of oil
- 2 tablespoons of mustard
- Paprika powder
- Salt and pepper

NUTRITIONAL VALUES **per serving**
Kcal
693
Protein
44.43 g
Fat

54.21 g
Carbohydrate

1. g

PREPARATION

1. Processing time about 30 minutes
2. Cooking / cooking time approx. 1 hour
3. Total time about 1 hour and 30 minutes
4. Finely chop the garlic cloves, onion, paprika and chives.
5. Mix the minced meat, eggs, mustard, tomato paste, salt, pepper and paprika powder.

1. Add the chopped vegetables, take half of the chives and mix. Then pour the mixture into a baking dish and distribute everything evenly. Bake inside the oven at 200 °c for 15 minutes.

1. Cut the remaining onions and peppers into large cubes. Mix the sour cream with the tomatoes and water until you get a homogeneous mixture. Season with salt and pepper.

1. After 15 minutes, take the mold out of the oven and spread the tomato mixture on top. Then distribute the remaining vegetables and finally sprinkle with cheese. Bake in the oven for another 45 minutes. Serve later.

18
KIDA LOW CARB GYROS PIZZA

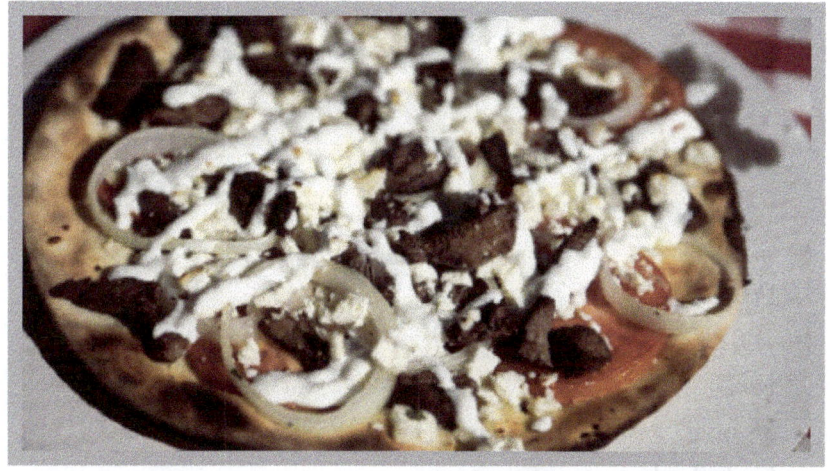

15 MINUTES.
Normal
781 kcal

INGREDIENTS

3 servings

- 500 g of beef gyros
- 1 courgette
- 1 bell pepper
- Eighth cherry tomato
- 3 eggs)
- 200 g of cottage cheese
- 125 g of grated cheese for topping
- 75 g of grated cheese with gratin
- Sea salt and pepper
- Cayenne pepper
- 1 teaspoon of coconut oil for frying

Nutritional values per serving

Kcal

781

Protein

71.84 g

Fat

49.99 g

Carbohydrate

1. g

PREPARATION

KETO PIZZA

1. Processing time about 15 minutes
2. Cooking / cooking time approx. 30 minutes
3. Total time about 45 minutes
4. Preheat the oven to 220 ° c.

1. Place the eggs, grated cheese and granulated cream cheese in a bowl and mix. Cut the courgettes into cubes, wash and cut the peppers into cubes, wash and quarter the tomatoes. Add the vegetables to the egg mixture, season with sea salt, pepper, and cayenne pepper and mix well. Place the mixture on a baking sheet lined with parchment paper and distribute it evenly. Put the pan in the oven for 20 minutes.

1. Melt the coconut oil in the pan and fry the gyros. Place the meat on the finished base, sprinkle with grated cheese and place the pizza in the oven for another 5 - 10 minutes, until the cheese is golden.

19

LOW CARB PIZZA MADE WITH AN EGG CURD DOUGH

KETO PIZZA

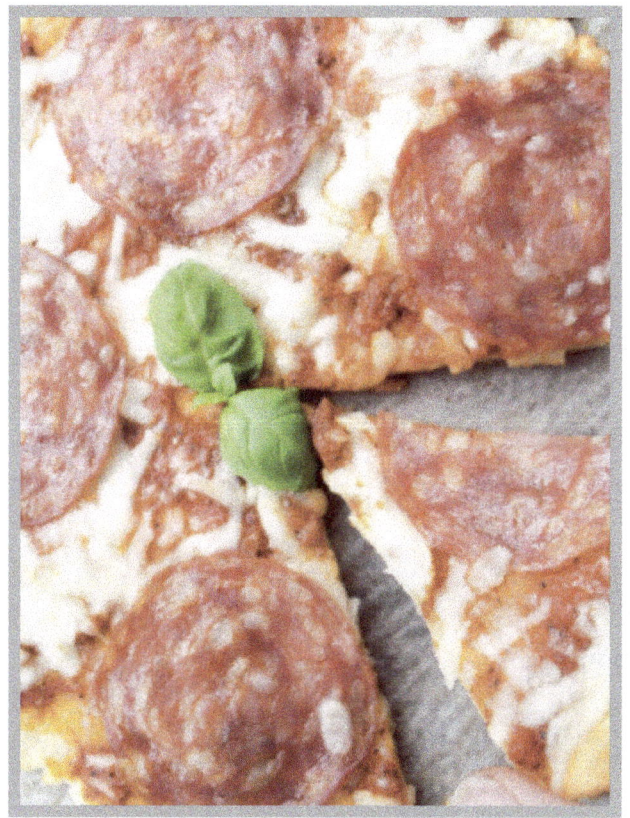

10 MINUTES.

Normal

345 kcal

INGREDIENTS

3 servings

- 3 eggs)
- 3 tablespoons cottage cheese
- 1 pinch of salt
- 1 pinch of pepper

- 150 ml tomato (s), success
- 2 tablespoons tomato sauce, light
- 100 g of grated cheese
- 8 slices of cooked ham

Nutritional values per serving
Kcal
3. 4. 5
Protein
32.72 g
Fat
20.48 g
Carbohydrate
7.10 g

PREPARATION

1. Working time approx. 10 minutes.
2. Cooking time / cooking time approx. 30 minutes
3. Total time approx. 40 minutes
4. Preheat the oven to 180 ° c with a fan. Line two baking sheets with parchment paper.

1. Separate the eggs. Mix the yolks with the cottage cheese, salt and pepper, beat the whites until they are

compact and add them to the mixture of cottage cheese and yolks.

1. Form 8 small pizzas, arrange on the baking tray and bake for 20 minutes at 180 °c.

1. Mix the tomatoes and tomato sauce, spread on the pizzas, decorate with ham and cheese and bake for another 10 minutes until the cheese melts.

20
LOW CARB PIZZA WITH BAKED POTATOES AND EGG WHITES

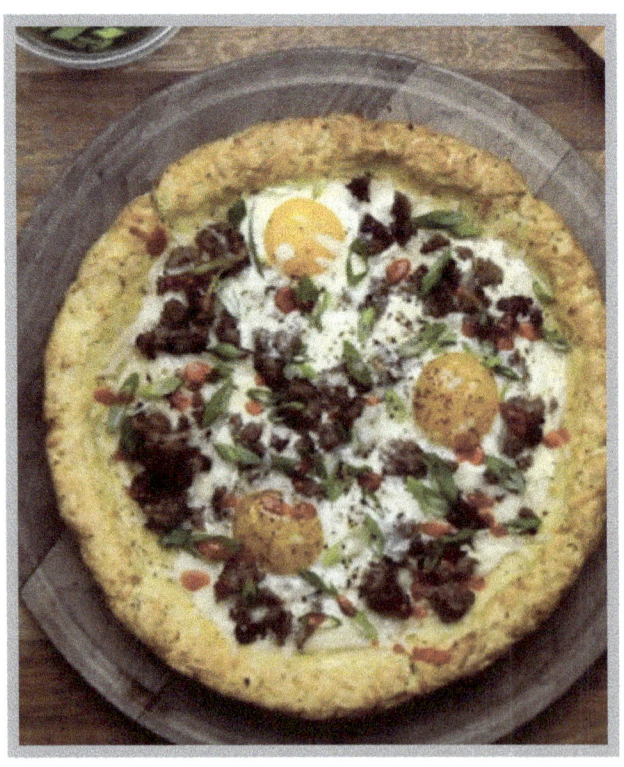

KETO PIZZA

30 MINUTES.

Normal

INGREDIENTS

1 servings

- 300 g potatoes
- 80 g spelled flour
- 80g protein powder (baked protein)
- 30 g spelled bran
- 20 g psyllium husk
- 2 teaspoons of yeast to tartare
- 30 ml oil
- N. B. Water
- Nb tomatoes, it happened
- N. B. Pizza topping
- N.b. Salami
- N. B. Ham
- N.b. Grated cheese

PREPARATION

1. Working time approx. 30 minutes.
2. Cooking time / cooking time approx. 30 minutes
3. Total time approx. 1 hour
4. Sxrape the potatoes, cut them into small pieces and cook them until soft (i cooked them in the microwave

for about 10 minutes). Let cool a little and mash with a fork.

1. Now add the flour, yeast protein, spelled bran, psyllium husks, baking powder, and oil to the potatoes and mix well. And then add a little water to form a smooth dough. Spread the dough out on a parchment lined baking sheet or roll it out thinly.

1. Place the second rack from the bottom at 220 ° c for about 15 minutes.

1. Brush the base with the tomato sauce and sprinkle with the pizza topping. Top with salami, ham, and shredded cheese (or seasoning of your choice). Make a bake for another 15 minutes at the same temperature on the second rack from the bottom.

21
LOW CARB PIZZA TUNA

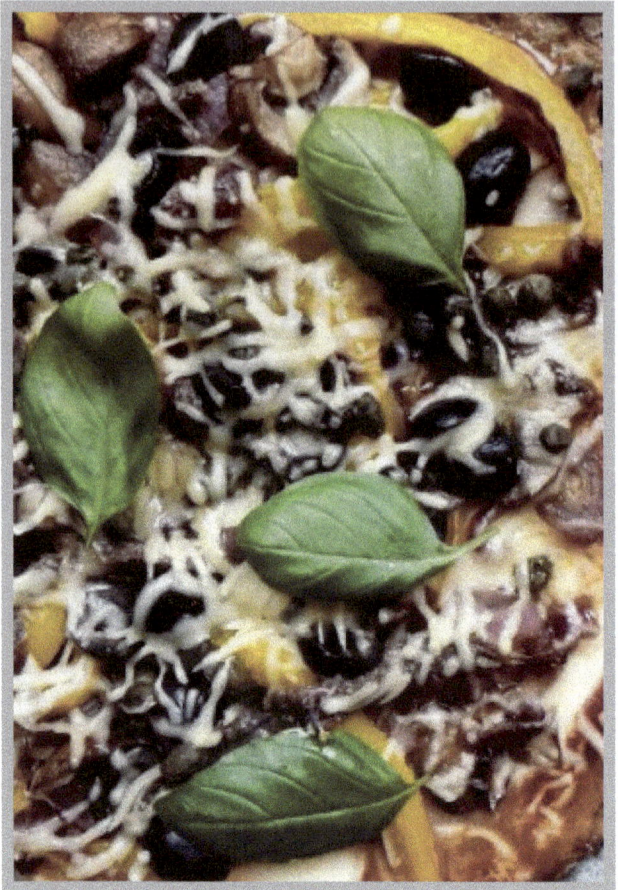

10 MINUTES.

Normal

INGREDIENTS

1 servings

- 1 can of tuna in its own juice
- 2 eggs)
- 2 tablespoons tomato (i), right

- 1 handful of cheese for pizza
- 5 slices of chicken breast fillets or ham
- 1 handful of icing sugar)

PREPARATION

1. Working time approx. 10 minutes.
2. Cooking time / cooking time approx. 15 minutes
3. Total time approx. 25 minutes
4. For the dough, beat the two eggs together. Chop and mix the tuna until only a few pieces of tuna remain. Place on a round parchment paper lined baking sheet and bake in a preheated oven (air circulation 170-180 degrees) for 10 minutes.

1. Then take it out and sprinkle the tomatoes on top. Put the rest of the ingredients on the pizza and bake for another 5 minutes.

22
LOW CARB PIZZA MOZZARELLA

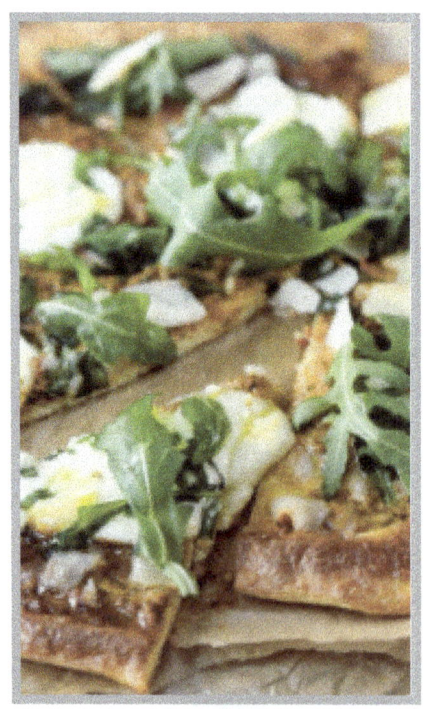

KETO PIZZA

30 MINUTES.
Easy
2665 kcal

INGREDIENTS

1 servings

- 600 g of mozzarella
- 100 g of grated parmesan cheese
- 100 g of cream cheese
- 3 eggs)
- 1 can of tomatoes, cut into pieces, 425 ml
- Salt and pepper
- Topping for pizza
- North. B. Pepper
- 4. Mushrooms
- 50 g of smoked turkey breast

PREPARATION

1. Processing time about 30 minutes
2. Cooking time / cooking approx. 45 minutes
3. Total time about 1 hour and 15 minutes
4. Brush a pan with oil and cover with mozzarella cut into thin slices. Save the remaining mozzarella for garnish.

1. Mix the cream cheese, eggs and parmesan cheese and pour over the mozzarella.

1. Bake the pizza dough at 180 ° c for about 30 minutes. Remove from the oven, cover with the spiced tomato pieces, the chopped pepper, the finely chopped mushrooms, the turkey breast cubes and the remaining mozzarella slices and cover for about 10-15 minutes until golden brown.

1. 2665 kcal per serving

23
LOW CARB PIZZA

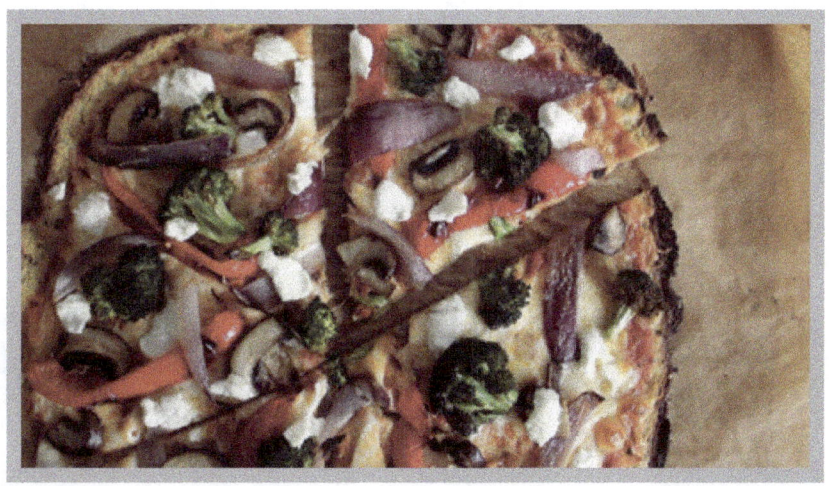

15 MINUTES.
   Easy

INGREDIENTS

1 servings

- 2 cups of cottage cheese
- 4 m eggs.
- 1 packet of gouda, grated, approx. 200 g
- 30 g of chopped almonds
- 1 large pepper
- 1 pack of cooked ham, approx. 100 grams
- 1 pack of salami, approx. 100 grams
- 2 large tomatoes)
- 1 pinch of salt
- 1 teaspoon of oregano
- 1 teaspoon of pizza topping

PREPARATION

1. Processing time about 15 minutes
2. Cooking time / cooking approx. 35 minutes
3. Total time about 50 minutes
4. Combine the ricotta, eggs and almonds in a food processor or standard hand mixer with a whisk.

1. Cut the rest of the ingredients, in my case peppers, cooked ham, salami and tomatoes, with a knife. You can also use other ingredients for the filling.

1. Now add all the finely chopped ingredients and spices with the batter mixture to the bowl. I always use pizza topping, oregano and some salt, you have to try it to see how best it is. Also put the gouda in the bowl and mix everything properly so that everything mixes very well and you have an even batter.

1. Extend the dough evenly on a baking sheet lined with baking paper so that all the baking paper is covered with it.

1. Bake in a preheated oven at 200 ° c for about 35 minutes. You can tell the pizza is ready when the edge, which is usually thinner, turns brown.

24
LOW CARB VEGETARIAN PIZZA

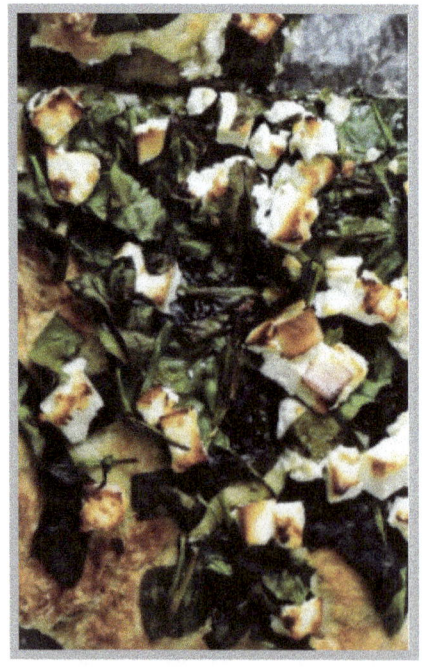

20 MINUTES.

KETO PIZZA

Normal

INGREDIENTS

1 servings

- 1 cauliflower, approx. 1 kg
- 8 large eggs
- 800 g of grated cheese
- 4 cups of fresh cream cheese
- 2 large onions (m)
- 3 peppers
- Salt and pepper
- It can grease

PREPARATION

1. Processing time about 20 minutes
2. Cooking / cooking time about 40 minutes
3. Total time about 1 hour
4. For the base, clean and grate the raw cauliflower. Then mix the grater with the eggs and 400 g of grated cheese.spray this mixture evenly on a greased baking sheet.

1. Bake the lower part in a preheated oven at 180 ° c high / low or in a convection oven at 160 ° c for 25

minutes.

1. In the meantime, peel and chop the onions and peppers for the filling. Then mix with the crème fraîche and the rest of the cheese. Season the mixture with salt and pepper.

1. Spread the filling on the pre-cooked base and bake the pizza for another 15 minutes.

TIP: if you don't want a vegetarian pizza, spread the ham cubes on the pizza before continuing to cook.

25
LOW CARB FLOURLESS PIZZA

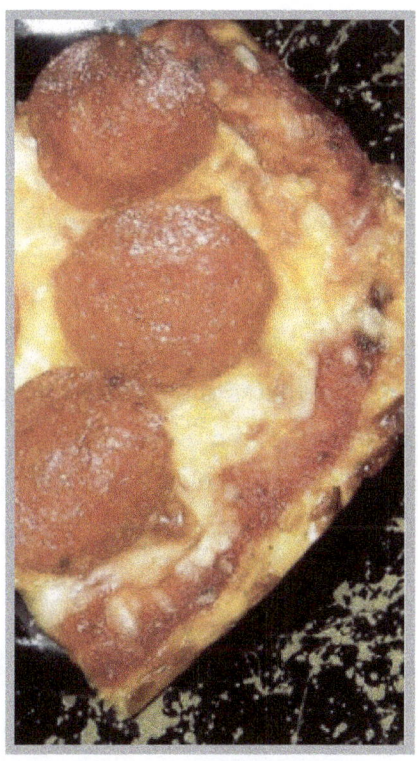

10 MINUTES.

Easy

277 kcal

INGREDIENTS

1 servings

- 60 g low-fat cottage cheese
- 60 g of lightly grated cheese
- 1 egg (s), size m.
- 3 tablespoons tomato paste
- Salt
- Pepper
- A little basil
- Some oregano

PREPARATION

1. Working time approx. 10 minutes.
2. Cooking time / cooking time approx. 25 minutes
3. Total time approx. 35 minutes
4. Preheat oven to 180 ° c (200 ° c top / bottom heat).

1. Mix the low-fat curd, cheese, and egg well in a bowl.

1. Spread the "dough" on a parchment paper lined baking sheet (pizza is slightly smaller than frozen pizza). Pre-bake the skillet over medium heat for 15 minutes.

1. Take out the tray.

1. Blend the tomato paste with a little water, salt, pepper, oregano and basil and season to taste.
2. Spread the dough with the tomato sauce and decorate to taste. Then bake the pizza for another 10 minutes.

1. The caloric value of 277 kcal per serving only refers to the dough without topping.

26
LOW CARB KETO PIZZA FLAMBÉ BUNS

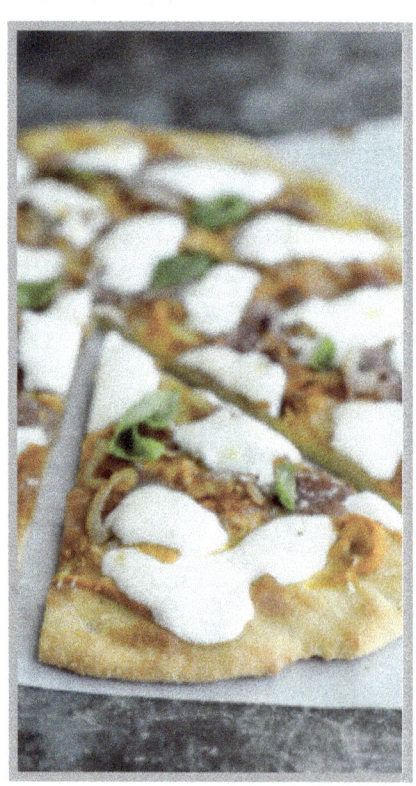

15 MINUTES.
Easy

INGREDIENTS

1 servings

- 2 eggs)
- 120 g low-fat cottage cheese
- 130 g of grated cheese, lightly
- 100 g crème fraîche, alternatively crème lègére
- 1 bunch of chives (m)
- 50 g of diced ham
- N.b. Salt and pepper
- 1 tablespoon of herbs or fresh cream of herbs

PREPARATION

1. Working time approx. 15 minutes
2. Rest time of about five minutes.
3. Cooking time / cooking time approx. 30 minutes
4. Total time approx. 50 minutes
5. For the base, mix the low-fat quark with the eggs and 80g cheese and stir until smooth. Season with a little salt and pepper.

1. Place the liquid mixture on a parchment lined baking sheet and distribute it evenly. One serving is more or less enough for one skillet, but it can vary slightly depending on the size of the oven. As is usual with a flambé tart, the mixture can be spread very thinly.

1. Bake in preheated 175 ° c high / low or 160 ° c convection oven for about 15 minutes on the middle shelf until a light golden brown color appears. Do not bake for a long time as the dough will return to the oven after filling. If small bubbles form, put them in with a fork to keep the bottom nice and smooth. As soon as the desired brown color is achieved, take the dough out of the oven and let it cool for about 5 minutes.
2. Tip: during this time, i briefly remove the base from the parchment paper, as experience has shown that it can be better processed later.

1. Spread the fresh cream over the dough. If you like, you can season a little with salt and pepper. Sprinkle with the sliced chives, ham and the remaining 50g cheese.

1. Return to the oven on the center rack for about 15

minutes, until the cheese is melted and lightly browned.

1. If desired, you can eat it as a low carb flambé tart or let the cake cool briefly and carefully roll it up with parchment paper and cut into small pieces.

1. Depending on the ingredients used, the snacks only contain around 6g of carbohydrates.

1. Of course, you can also add flambé cake or sandwiches to taste. Here, for example, the variant with salmon is really excellent in terms of taste.

27

LOW CARB PIZZA WITH MEAT AND ONION TOPPINGS

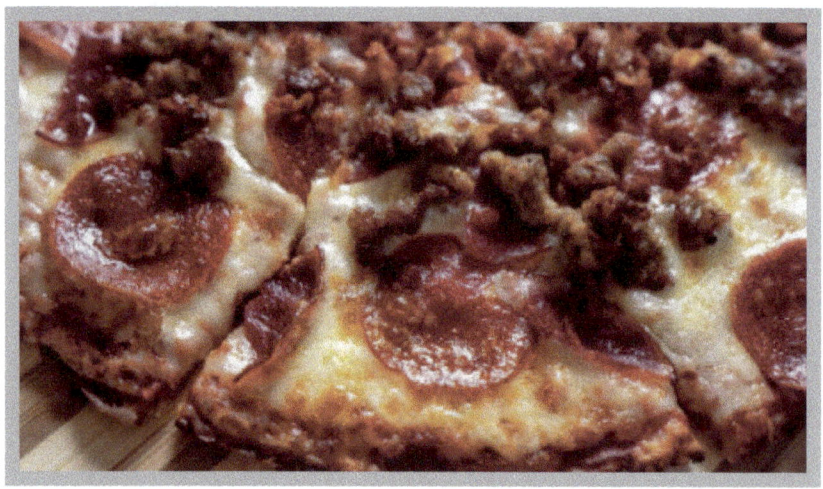

10 MINUTES.
 Easy

INGREDIENTS

KETO PIZZA

1 servings

- 1 pkg. Pizza dough, low carb from the refrigerated shelf (pizza dough)
- 100 g of beef tenderloin from the day before
- 1 small onion
- 75 g cheese for pizza
- N. B. Clarified butter

PREPARATION

1. Working time approx. 10 minutes.
2. Cooking time / cooking time approx. 25 minutes
3. Total time approx. 35 minutes
4. Preheat the oven to 220 ° c (top / bottom heat). Pre-bake the dough according to the manufacturer's instructions.

1. Finely chop the meat and onion. Fry both briefly in clarified butter. Spread the meat and onion mixture over the dough and sprinkle with cheese. Bake in the oven for 10 minutes.

28
LOW CARB PIZZA WITH PORK NECK AND RATATOUILLE

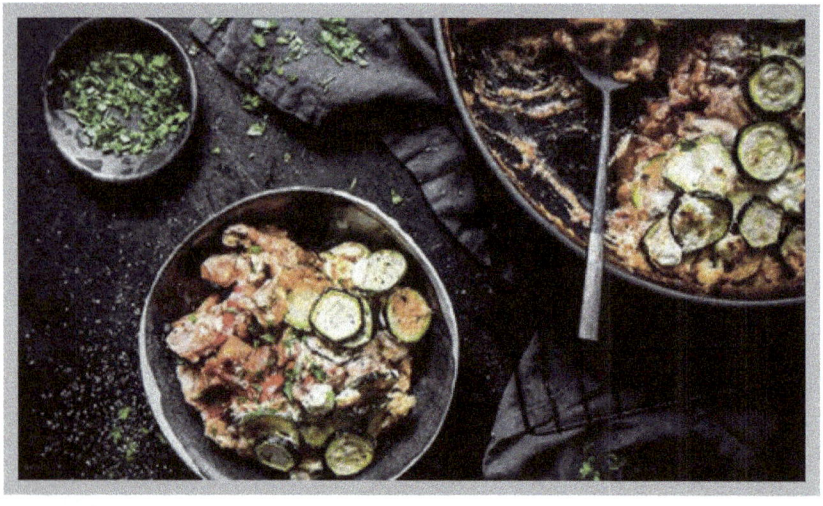

30 MINUTES.
   Easy

INGREDIENTS

KETO PIZZA

1 Servings

- 1 package pizza dough, low carb, from the refrigerated shelf (pizza dough)
- 1 smaller pork neck
- 5 tbsp, heaped vegetables (ratatouille) from the day before
- 4 tbsp tomato sauce
- 2 chili
- 1 small onion (noun)
- N. B. Clarified butter
- N. B. Cheese, grated

PREPARATION

1. Working time approx. 20 minutes
2. Cooking / baking time approx. 25 minutes
3. Total time approx. 45 minutes
4. Pre-heat oven to 220 degrees celsius (top/bottom heat). Preheat the oven to 350°f and bake the dough according to the package directions.

1. Slice the onion and chillies into thin rings. Pork neck is cut into cubes and fried in clarified butter. Add the vegetables and cook for a few minutes. On the dough, spread the tomato sauce first, then the meat mixture.

1. Top with onion and chili, as well as grated cheese if desired. Preheat the oven to 350°f and bake for 10 minutes.

29
KETO PIZZA DOUGH

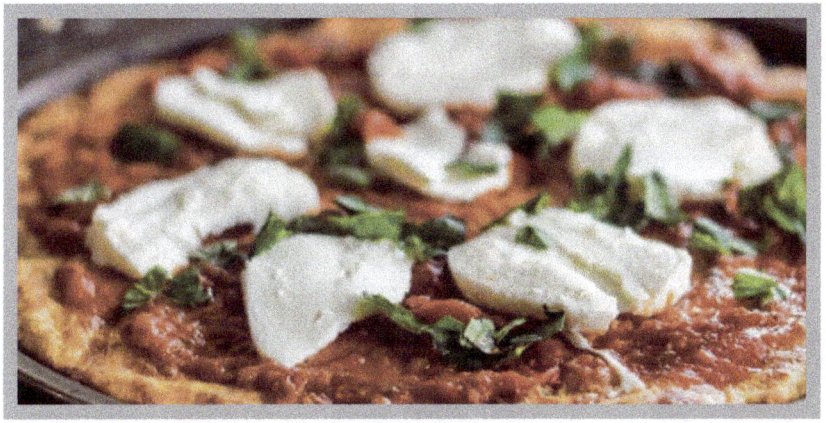

20 MINUTES.
  Servings 8
  Easy

INGREDIENTS

- 2 cups Mozzarella cheese shredded
- 1 oz cream cheese
- 1 cup almond flour super-fine
- 1 egg
- 1 tsp baking powder
- 1 tsp Italian seasoning
- ½ cup Low-carb tomato sauce
- 4 oz fresh Mozzarella
- 4 basil leaves fresh, torn

PREPARATION

Heat up your oven to 425 degrees Fahrenheit and put a pizza stone in the middle rack.

In a glass cup, combine the shredded Mozzarella and cream cheese and microwave for 45 seconds. Mix in the remaining ingredients for the low-carb crust thoroughly.

Apply a thin coating of olive oil to your hands and put the dough on a large sheet of parchment paper. Place another layer of parchment paper on top of the dough and flatten it out slightly. Using a rolling pin, roll out the dough to a thickness of 14 inches. If you want to help shape the dough, you can do so with your hands.

If you have one, use it to move the pizza dough to the hot pizza plate. Bake for five minutes on one hand, then flip and bake for another five minutes on the other. Remove from the oven and top with your favorite keto-friendly toppings.

Bake for an additional five minutes or until the cheese topping is brown and bubbly.

www.ingramcontent.com/pod-product-compliance
Lightning Source LLC
Chambersburg PA
CBHW071116030426
42336CB00013BA/2104